HOMIAN EMMANUEL TAHI
Eboi EHUI

RAPID EVALUATION OF CONDOM USE (ERUP 2021)

HOMIAN EMMANUEL TAHI
Eboi EHUI

RAPID EVALUATION OF CONDOM USE (ERUP 2021)

EVALUATION OF AVAILABILITY, ACCESSIBILITY AND USE OF CONDOMS

Imprint

Any brand names and product names mentioned in this book are subject to trademark, brand or patent protection and are trademarks or registered trademarks of their respective holders. The use of brand names, product names, common names, trade names, product descriptions etc. even without a particular marking in this work is in no way to be construed to mean that such names may be regarded as unrestricted in respect of trademark and brand protection legislation and could thus be used by anyone.

Cover image: www.ingimage.com

This book is a translation from the original published under ISBN 978-620-6-71639-6.

Publisher:
Sciencia Scripts
is a trademark of
Dodo Books Indian Ocean Ltd. and OmniScriptum S.R.L publishing group

120 High Road, East Finchley, London, N2 9ED, United Kingdom
Str. Armeneasca 28/1, office 1, Chisinau MD-2012, Republic of Moldova, Europe
Printed at: see last page
ISBN: 978-620-7-90730-4

TABLE OF CONTENTS

THANKS

The Programme National de Lutte contre le Sida (PNLS) would like to thank all the member organisations of the Groupe Technique de Travail sur le Condom (GTTCCP) for their facilitation of this evaluation.

It would also like to thank all the Regional and Departmental Directorates of Health, Public Hygiene and Universal Health Coverage, which were covered by the evaluation, for the quality of the welcome given to the data collection teams and for their very qualitative facilitation.

*Special thanks go to Professor **EHUI Eboi,** Director of the National AIDS Control Programme and all the staff of the NACP for their invaluable support in making this study a success.*

Our sincere thanks go to the community leaders of the key populations and to the various managers of the Non-Governmental Organisations (NGOs) implementing HIV prevention and care activities for the key populations.

Not forgetting also the various people in charge of the hot spots in the localities covered by the mobilisation assessment.

To all of you, thank you very much for your invaluable contributions, which made it possible t o successfully collect the data for this evaluation.

INVESTIGATORS AND INSTITUTIONAL AFFILIATIONS

Ministry of Health, Public Hygiene and Universal Health Coverage, Côte d'Ivoire

- ***National AIDS Control Programme (PNLS)***

The PNLS is commissioning this study.

- ***Pr EHUI Eboi***, *Director-Coordinator of the PNLS, Principal Investigator, Tel : +225 77 19 27 05 / 05 06 28 66 ; Email : docehui@yahoo.fr eehui2@hotmail.com*

- ***Ms N'DA Viviane,*** *Head of Research at PNLS, Co-Investigator, Tel: +225 07 99 08 93, Email: vivinda@yahoo.fr*

Dr TAHI Homian Emmanuel, *Doctor, Technical Assistant, STI Management at the PNLS, Co-investigator, telephone: +225.05 84 53 35 52 ; E-mail: tahi.emmanuel@pnls-ci.com*

- ***Mr KONE Foungnigué,*** *Assistant Evaluation and Research Officer, Research Department, PNLS, Co-Investigator, Tel: +225 07 98 90 22 / 84 53 15 03; Email: konefoungniguesimon@gmail.com*

- ***Global Fund***

The Global Fund to Fight Tuberculosis, Malaria and HIV/AIDS is the sponsor of this study.

IMPLEMENTATION TEAM EVALUATION

Study coordinator

*- **Dr TAHI Homian Emmanuel**, Doctor, Technical Assistant, STI Care at the PNLS, telephone: +225.05 84 53 35 52; E-mail: tahi.emmanuel@pnls-ci.com .*

Statisticians pool and data collection tool design

*- **Mr DIAKITE Ali;** Monitoring and Evaluation Assistant, PNLS, Email: diakite.ali@pnls-ci.com, Tel: 05 46 73 52 77*

*- **Mr KONE Foungnigué,** Assistant Evaluation and Research Officer, Research Department, PNLS, Email: kone.fougnigue@pnls-ci.com , Tel: +225 07 98 90 22 / 84 53 15 03*

-

Data collection staff

N°	FULL NAME	FUNCTION	STRUCTURE
1	Mrs ADON ALEXANDRINE	Midwife	PNLS
2	Dr. TAHI H. EMMANUEL	Doctor	PNLS
3	Ms CHERIF AWA	Programme Manager	ROCPCI
4	Dr. KOFFI ASSIE LEON	Pharmacist	PNLS
5	MR OUATTARA OUMAR	Monitoring and evaluation	AIMAS
6	Dr AHOUA P. Adingra	Prevention consultant	PNLS
7	Mr ASSOUMOU Noel	Evaluator follow-up	PNLS
8	Dr LADE Jacquelin Gémie	Programme Manager	AIBEF
9	BEUGRE Claudy Yvonne	Midwife	CIVIL SOCIETY

DEFINITION OF SOME CONCEPTS

Requirements: Number of products and services needed to cover a given market.

Unsatisfied needs: Demand for products and services exceeds supply / set of expectations of a person or institution not taken into account

Unit price: monetary value of the unit of a product

Distribution: All the activities involved in managing customer orders and making products available to customers. These operations include storing products in suitable conditions, managing them according to clearly defined rules, recording and processing customer orders, dispatching products, transporting them and delivering them to customers.

Distribution channel: This covers all the distribution channels for a product. The aim is to highlight the route taken by a product from the producer to the consumer, including all potential intermediaries (or, conversely, the absence of intermediaries). It is not unusual to differentiate between short and long distribution channels. Short distribution channels focus on a direct relationship between producer and consumer (limiting the number of intermediaries and favouring local distribution channels). Long distribution channels involve intermediaries (wholesalers, traders, distributors, etc.) in the marketing of a product between a producer and a consumer.

Dispensing: The process of delivering prescribed pharmaceutical products to the customer. It must ensure and promote the effective and rational use of products.

Procurement: All the operations involved in forecasting quantities and costs, planning deliveries and acquiring pharmaceutical products.

Market share: The market share of a product, service or company in a given market is the percentage of its sales in that market compared with the total sales of that product by all companies. It is used to situate or compare companies in the market, to determine their position and that of their products and services in relation to competing companies.

Total Market Approach (TMA): A process by which providers and financiers from all sectors (public, social marketing and private) build a common strategic framework to improve **equity, efficiency** and **sustainability of** the health system in order to maximise the use of condoms and lubricant gels. The AMT uses the conceptual framework and tools of the total market system to: (i) understand the underlying causes of persistent problems in condom and gel use; (ii) identify system-wide interventions to mitigate the challenges; and (iii) launch initiatives that promote sustainable change.

Availability: All the activities aimed at making a product or service available to the various population groups, whatever the geographical area.

Accessibility: All activities aimed at making it easier for people to acquire a product or services, whatever their geographical location.

Equity: A concept (according to the WHO) that is defined as "the absence of unjust and avoidable or redressable differences in health between populations or groups defined socially, economically, demographically or geographically". Equity in health is an ethical principle founded on the basic notions of distributive justice. This concept is closely linked to the principle of human rights and equal opportunities for all people to enjoy good health.

Coverage of requirements: The ratio of production data to objects (targets)

Sexual relations at risk: All sexual relations with a non-cohabiting partner, non-marital partner, occasional partner, boyfriend, client.

SUMMARY

The highly ambitious NSP 2021-2025 aims to achieve a 90% rate of systematic condom use during high-risk sex among sexually active people, compared with 44.6% in 2018 (CIPHIA 2018).

To this end, the Ministry of Health, Public Hygiene and Universal Health Coverage, through the PNLS, has set up a surveillance system as part of the total market approach in sentinel towns, where it has carried out a rapid assessment of the availability, accessibility and use of condoms. The aim is to assess the distribution chain and the use of condoms and lubricant gels.

Methodology: This is a descriptive quantitative analysis based on an interview using a digital questionnaire sent to the players (wholesalers, semi-wholesalers and sales outlets in the vicinity of the hot spots) and users found in the hot spots.

Results: The following indicator data **were** obtained:

Availability: **In** 2021, the quantities of condoms distributed by the different sectors of the total market will be 5,294,200 (26%) free, 14,341 470 (71%) for social marketing and 581,815 (3%) for the private sector. Only 07 of the 30 towns assessed have coverage of needs ≥ 100%. These are the towns of Bondoukou (269%), Adzopé (161%), Abengourou (145%), Soubré (127%), Guiglo, etc. (124%), Daloa (101%) and Séguéla (100%).mAccessibility: 148 POS for 158 hotspots visited (ratio= 0.9). Of the 148 outlets visited, 91% were open 7 days a week, 64% remained open after midnight, 91% used the "pay by cash" option as a supply method and 84% had a permanent supply of condoms. The shops, which account for 60% of the outlets (97% open 7 days a week, 56% stay open after midnight and 90 % have permanent availability) and aprons representing 19% of outlets (86% are open 7 days a week, 79% stay open after midnight and 79% have permanent availability). permanent availability) ensure that people have better access to condoms.

Use: All participants (1707) were sexually active and the average age at first sexual intercourse was 18 for the general population and 17 for the key populations, with condom use rates of 29% and 31% respectively. The rate of condom use at first sexual intercourse before the age of 15 (average age 13) is lower (21%), and still lower among boys (16%).

At last sexual intercourse, the condom use rate was 49% (men: 53%). women: 42%) for the general population. For key populations, this rate was 92% for TS, 83% for UD and TG and 75% for MSM.Multi-sex partnerships are observed in 65% of men and 50% of women.

I. BACKGROUND

Côte d'Ivoire, one of the countries most affected by HIV infection in West Africa, with a prevalence rate of 2.1% (SPECTRUM 2021), has committed to the global initiative to eliminate AIDS by 2030 through its national strategic plan (NSP 2021-2025) to combat STIs, HIV and AIDS [1].
Various UNAIDS models indicate that this initiative can only be achieved through the deployment of combined prevention interventions, of which condoms are a key component [2].

The highly ambitious NSP aims for the rate of systematic condom use during risky sex among sexually active people to be 90% by 2025 [1], compared with 44.6% in 2018 (CIPHIA 2018).To meet people's condom needs, the total market is made up of three segments: firstly, the free segment, led by the National AIDS Control Programme (PNLS); secondly, the social marketing segment, led by AIMAS (Agence Ivoirienne de Marketing Social); and thirdly, the commercial segment, which brings together the majority of players [3]. Achieving the NSP 2021-2025 objective requires the implementation of programmatic interventions that firstly ensure better availability of condoms, secondly improve their accessibility to priority populations and thirdly encourage their use during risky sexual relations.To this end, the Ministry of Health, Public Hygiene and Universal Health Coverage, through the PNLS, is setting up a system to monitor the availability, accessibility and use of condoms as part of the total market approach in selected sentinel towns.It is in this context that the NACP has organised a rapid assessment of condom use, thanks to the financial support of the Global Fund under NFM3, through its 2021 missions to supervise stakeholders and conduct biannual audits of data from sentinel surveillance sites.

II.OBJECTIVES

II.1. General objective

To assess the distribution chain and the use of condoms and lubricant gels.

II.2. Specific objectives

- Assess the availability of condoms and lubricant gels in sentinel towns;
- Evaluate access to condoms and lubricant gels for priority populations;
- Evaluate the use of condoms and lubricating gels;

- Formulate recommendations to address the shortcomings identified.

<h1 align="center">III. EVALUATION METHODOLOGY</h1>

This rapid assessment is based on a descriptive quantitative analysis by interview using a digital questionnaire, and on the collection of distribution data using district pharmacy management tools.

1. Location

1.1. Selection criteria

The methodology adopted is that of reasoned choices based on the 2020 STI incidence data and the 2017-2018 CIPHIA condom use data.

The cities selected had both a higher incidence of STIs than the national level (23.3%) and a lower rate of condom use than the national level (44.6%).

1.2. Selected cities

The 36 towns identified/selected as sentinel towns are : BEOUMI, BOUAKE, BUYO, DALOA, DIVO, GUIGLO, KANI, KATIOLA, KORO, KOUNAHIRI, MANKONO, OUANINOU, SAKASSOU, SAN-PEDRO, SEGUELA, TABOU, TOUBA, YAMOUSSOUKRO, BONDOUKOU, AGBOVILLE, BANGOLO, OUANGOLODOUGOU, BOUAFLE, DUEKOUE, GAGNOA, ISSA, DAOUKRO, ABENGOUROU, AGNIBILEKRO, OUME, ODIENNE, ADZOPE, KORHOGO, SOUBRE, DANANE AND MAN.

2. Target population

By type of heading, these are :

• Availability of inputs :

o wholesalers and semi-wholesalers in the social and private marketing sector;

o pharmacies in the health districts for free;

• Accessibility of condoms: retailers in the vicinity of hot spots;

- Condom use: people present at the hot spots at the time of collection.

population	Inclusion criteria	Non-inclusion criteria
Wholesalers and Semi-wholesalers	Being located in sentinel towns Wholesale and semi-wholesale of condoms and lubricating gels Belong to the public sector or the social marketing sector or the private sector	-Retail condoms and lubricant gels
Retailers	Retail sale of condoms and lubricant gels Be located in the vicinity of hot	- Be a wholesale distributor of condoms and lubricant gels, and half-wholesale
Use of condoms	Be male or female, aged 15 or over Being sexually active Be present at the identified hot-spot at the time of collection	Be male or female and under 15 years of age Not consenting to take part in the survey Not to have already been surveyed

3. Sampling

For availability, the study took into account all wholesalers and semi-wholesalers in each locality. For accessibility, only retailers in the vicinity of hot-spots were taken into account. A minimum of 10 people were interviewed for each hot spot identified.

4. Collection tool

A single digitalised questionnaire for standardised individual interviews has been developed in French to collect data. The questionnaire has three interfaces relating to the sub-groups of the study population: one for wholesalers and semi-wholesalers relating to availability, one for retailers relating to accessibility and one for the condom users in relation to the use of condoms during risky sex. This is a structured questionnaire, pre-coded for certain response modes and containing instructions for correct completion.

5. Data collection process

Information letters and the Terms of Reference (ToR) for this rapid assessment were sent to the Regional and Departmental Health Directors of the towns concerned before the data collection.Nine (09) evaluators from the CCP-TWG were trained in data collection procedures and tools. Three teams of three evaluators were deployed for data collection.

Data collection took place from 05 to 18 August and from 05 to 20 December 2021 with the support of resource persons provided by AIMAS (for data collection with wholesalers and semi-wholesalers) and by community-based organisations (CBOs) working with key populations (for data collection at hot spots).

The private sector has not been able to provide resource persons to collect from other wholesalers and semi-wholesalers not supplied by AIMAS.

All those interviewed about condom use received condoms in accordance with current distribution guidelines[1] . All the sites visited were geolocated.

6. Ethical considerations

Rules for checking the consistency of the data collected have been set up in the ODK questionnaire so that the teams correct as many errors as possible before transmission to the server.

7. Data quality control

The data quality assurance process includes checking the questionnaire for internal consistency: examining response errors, missing information, checking limits, logical checks, etc. Rules for checking the consistency of the data collected have been set up in the digitised questionnaire so that the teams can correct any aberrant/inconsistent data in situ before transmitting it to the server.

8. Data entry, reconciliation, validation

All variables were labelled with value codes. Qualitative responses to open-ended questions were coded, as were responses of type
"Other: specify". The data was entered using EPI data software.

9. Data confidentiality

All the data collected is entered into a protected database, accessible only by the PNLS. Only aggregated data is published. No structure/organisation/person can be identified from the data. Extraction files containing individual data by structure/organisation are stored in a locked location.

10. Data analysis

Data entered using EPI data was exported to the appropriate STATA software for descriptive analysis. This analysis highlighted retrospective condom and lubricant gel distribution data for the period January-June 2021.

IV. ANALYSIS OF RESULTS

1. Results general

During data collection, all 30 of the 36 towns sampled were visited. These visits were used to assess the availability and accessibility of condoms and lubricant gels, as well as condom use among people frequenting the hot spots (see table 1).

Table 1: Total number of facilities visited and participants interviewed

Availability	Accessibility		Use
	Hot spots	Where to buy	
33Pharmacies at	45 Close houses	89 Shops	
sanitary district	31 hotels	28 Aprons	
37 Wholesalers	58 Maquis	14 hotels	
66 Semi-wholesalers	13 Bars 08 Maquis-Bars 01 bistro 02 Space for	01 Coffee kiosks 02 Tobacco kiosks 02 Vending machines automatic	1707 people interviewed
	meeting	08 Private practices	
		02 Superettes	
		01 Maquis	
		01 Bistro	

The hotspots visited were dominated by maquis (37%), brothels (28%) and brothels (20%). The sales outlets in the vicinity of these hotspots where condom availability was assessed were mainly shops (60%), aprons (19%), brothels (9%) and private pharmacies (5%). Condom use was assessed in 1707 people.

2. Availability

The analysis of availability data covered the year 2021.

2.1. Sourcing

2.1.1. Ordering

Two indicators were used to assess the supply of products to facilities or product management points: orders and stock-outs.

A comparison is made between district pharmacies (free) and wholesalers and semi-wholesalers (social marketing and private sector) in terms of orders placed, orders fulfilled and stock-outs (see graph 1).

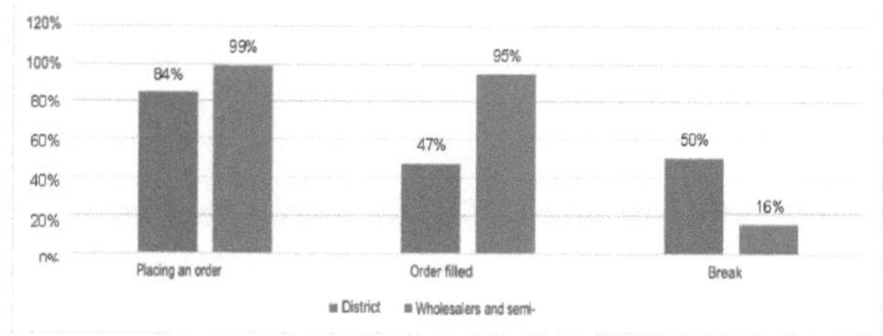

Graph 1: Comparison of orders and stock-outs between district pharmacies and wholesalers and semi-wholesalers

During 2021, 99% (94) of the wholesalers and semi-wholesalers evaluated placed orders and 95% (90) had their orders filled, compared with 84% (17/32) and 47% (14/32) respectively for district pharmacies.During the same period, stock-outs were observed in 16% of cases. (15) of wholesalers and semi-wholesalers compared with 50% (17) of district pharmacies.

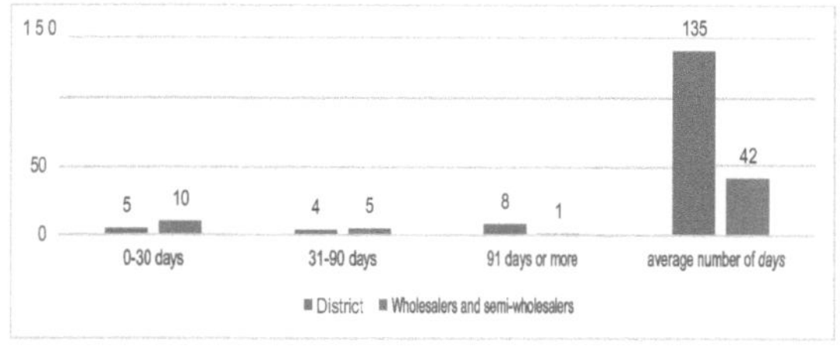

Graph 2: Number of days condoms were out of stock by market sector

District pharmacies were out of stock for an average of 135 days, compared with 42 days for wholesalers and semi-wholesalers.

2.1.2. Reasons for break-ups

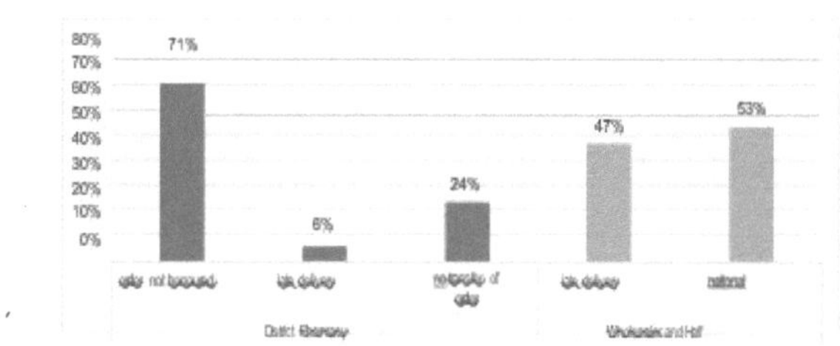

Graph 3: Reasons for stock shortages by market sector

The main reasons for stock-outs for district pharmacies are unfulfilled orders (71%) and failure to place an order (24%). For wholesalers and semi-wholesalers, the main reasons were national stock-outs (53%) and delivery delays (47%). It should be noted that AIMAS experienced a stock-out of the COMPLICE condom in January and February 2021.

2.2. Distribution

For distribution, the indicators assessed were the number of condoms distributed by market sector and coverage of needs by locality. The largest quantities of condoms distributed were in the towns of BONDOUKOU (2,779,140), BOUAKE (1,986,902), SOUBRE (1,906,040) and DALOA (1,876,389) and the lowest in the towns of KORO (7 500), OUANINOU (3,600), KOUNAHIRI (13,500) and OUME (15,600) (Cf. table 1in the appendix).

2.2.1. Condom distribution by sector of the market

In 2021, the quantities of condoms distributed by the different sectors of the total market are 5,294,200 (26%) for free, 14,341,470 (71%) for social marketing and 581,815 (3%) for the private sector (see table 1 in annex). The market is dominated by the social marketing sector in 18 towns, compared with 12 towns (OUANINOU and SAKASSOU) for free (see Graph 4).

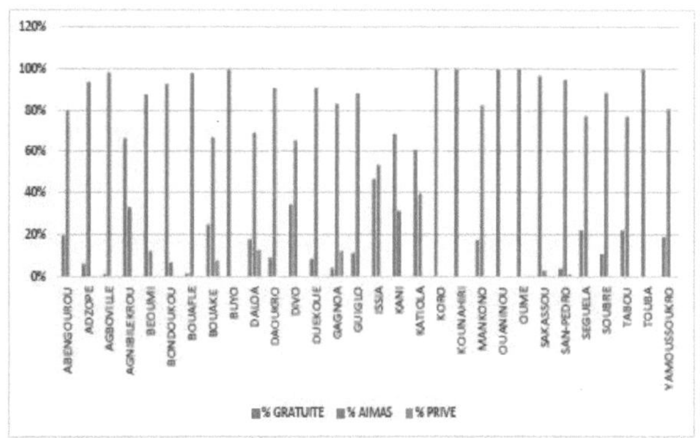

Graph 4: Shares of condom distribution by market sector

However, in 5 cities the marketing-social sector has no distribution data, and in all the sentinel cities the private sector is very poorly represented.

2.2.2. Coverage of needs

The UNAIDS/UNFPA quantification matrix was used to determine the condom needs of the towns visited in order to assess the coverage of the service offer in the first half of 2021 (see graph 5).

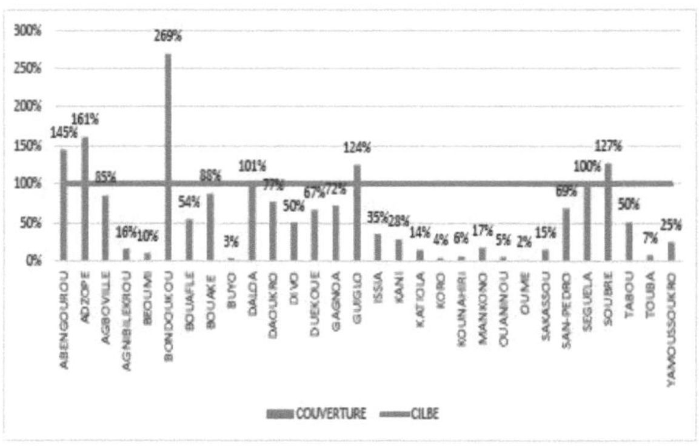

Graph 5: Coverage of condom needs at the end of June 2021

Only 07 towns and 2 towns out of the 30 assessed respectively exceed or come close to the expected target in terms of needs to be covered (100%): Bondoukou (269%), Adzopé (161%), Abengourou (145%), Soubré (127%), Guiglo (124%), Daloa (101%) and Séguéla (100%). However, 07 towns (Oumé, Buyo, Ouaninou, Koro, Béoumi, Touba and Kounahiri) have less than 10% coverage (see Graph 5).

3. Accessibility

For the accessibility assessment, the focus was on social marketing and private sector outlets in the vicinity of the hotspots.

3.1. Points of sale

The activities assessed by the sales outlets are the number of working days, the closing hours, the method of supply and the availability of condoms (see graph 6).

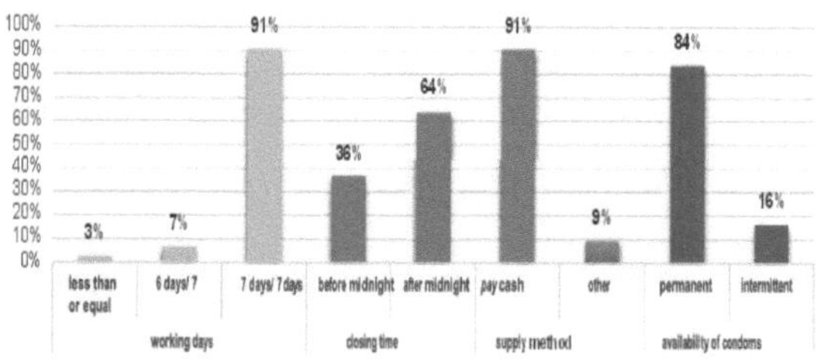

Graph 6: Breakdown of sales outlets by type of activity

Of the 148 sales outlets visited for 158 hot spots, 91% are open 7 days a week, 64% stay open after midnight, 91% use the "pay cash" option as a supply method and 84% have a permanent supply of condoms.Depot-sale" and "pay on credit" are the other procurement methods (9%). A comparison of these same indicators among the above-mentioned outlets is shown in graph 7.

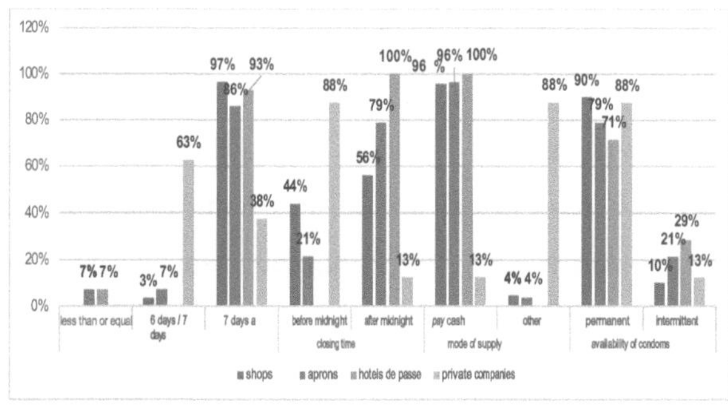

Figure 7: Breakdown of main sales outlets by type of activity

Boutiques, representing 60% of outlets in the vicinity of hot spots, were open 7 days a week in 97% of cases, had condoms available at all times in 90% of cases, but remained open after midnight in 56% of cases. In contrast, brothels, which accounted for 9% of outlets, were open 7 days a week in 93% of cases, had condoms permanently available in 71% of cases and remained open after midnight in 100% of cases, i.e. 24 hours a day.

3.2. Condom brands from l'AMT

During data collection, the different brands of condom found in the various sales outlets visited were recorded (see graph 8).

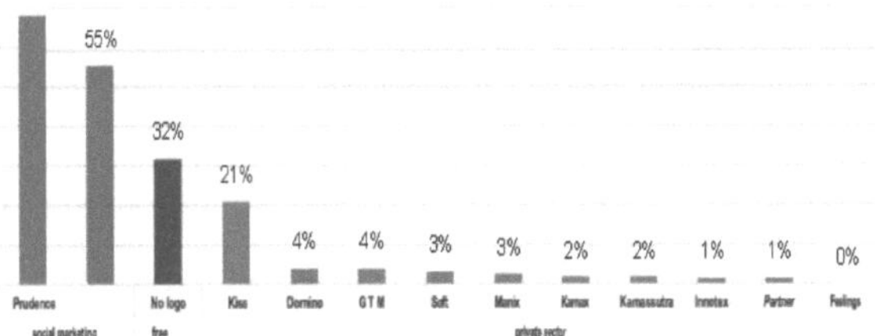

Figure 8: Representation of brands at the points of sale visited

The brands most represented in the outlets visited are **PRUDENCE** (68%), **COMPLICE** (55%), **NO-LOGO** (32%) and **KISS** (21%). The PRUDENCE and COMPLICE brands (from social marketing) and KISS (from the private sector) are distributed through wholesale distributors and pharmaceutical wholesalers. The least represented brands are from the private sector, mainly found in private pharmacies (see attached table) and distributed by pharmaceutical wholesalers.As regards the no-logo condom (intended for free distribution), under no circumstances should it be found at a point of sale, in accordance with current guidelines.The table below shows the different types of outlets involved in the sale of no-logo condoms.

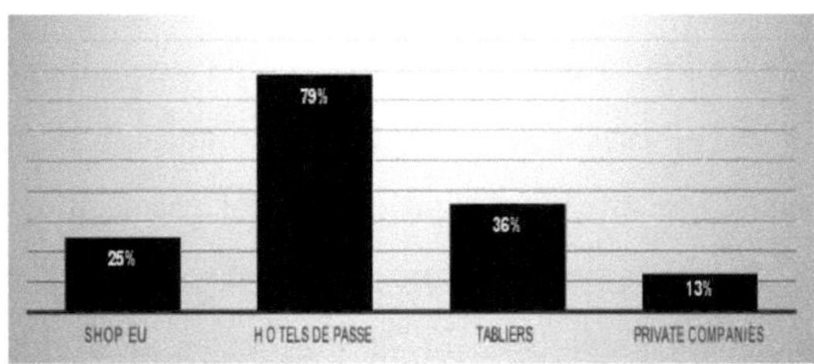

Graph 9: Representativeness o f sales outlets distributing no-logo condoms

Other condom brands (PROTECTOR, CONDOMS, HERO SON, LIVEX and TODAY) were also identified in 19 sales outlets, including 12 shops (see attached table).

4. Use

During data collection, the opinions of 1707 users were gathered on condoms (see table below).

Table 2: Breakdown of participants by population type and gender

By type of population	Workforce	By sub-group of populations	Workforce	By gender	Workforce
General	615 (36%)	15-24 years old	204 (33%)	Female	189 (31%)
		25 and over	411 (67%)	Male	426 (69%)
Key populations	1092 (64%)	TS	859 (79%)	Female	857 (78%)
		MSM	180 (16%)		
		UD	47 (4%)	Male	235 (22%)
		TG	6 (1%)		
Package	1707 (100%)			Female	1046 (61%)
				Male	661 (39%)

The general population was made up of 67% of people aged 25 and over; LTs represented 79% of the key populations and female respondents represented 61% of the total study population.

4.1. Sexual activities

Sexual activity was assessed in terms of first sexual intercourse, risky sexual intercourse in the last 12 months, frequency of sexual intercourse and multiple sexual partners.

4.1.1. First sex

Table 3: Average age and condom use at first intercourse

Features	Average age		Interval	Workforce	Percentage stating that a condom had been used	Workforce
GENERAL POPULATION						
WOMAN						
15-24 years old	17		10-21	79	35%	28
Aged 25-34	18		10-25	83	30%	25
35-49 years old	18		15-22	25	28%	7
50-64 years old	17		14-19	2	0%	0
Total women	17		10-25	189	32%	60
MEN						
15-24 years old		16	07-21	125	37%	46
Aged 25-34		17	08-29	157	29%	46
35-49 years old		19	14-37	123	17%	21
50-64 years old		20	14-25	15	27%	4
Total men		18	07-37	420	28%	117
TOTAL aged 15-64		18	07-37	609	29%	177
KEY POPULATION						
TS		17	07-28	859	29%	246
MSM		16	08-28	180	46%	82
UD		16	09-24	47	17%	8
TG		15	14-15	6	33%	2
Total KPs		17	07-28	1092	31%	338
ALL POPULATIONS		17	07-37	1701	30%	515
FIRST REPORT						
Before the age of 15	GIRL	13	07-14	196	24%	48
	BOY	13	07-14	126	16%	20
	Total	13	07-14	322	21%	68
At age 15 and over	WOMAN	17	15-28	850	30%	258
	MEN	18	15-37	535	36%	190
	Total	18	15-37	1385	32%	448
LEVEL OF EDUCATION						
Never been to school		17	09-37	467	22%	105
Preschool		17	15-22	5	20%	1
Primary		17	07-27	380	31%	119
Secondary		17	08-32	686	33%	225
Superior		17	07-25	142	42%	60

All participants (1707) were sexually active and the average age at first sexual intercourse was 18 for the general population and 17 for the key populations, with condom use rates of 29% and 31% respectively. Among the general population, the lowest rates of condom use (28% for females and 17% for males) were found in the 35-49 age group, and the highest (35% for females and 37% for males) in the 15-24 age group.Among key populations, condom use was lowest among DU (17%) and highest among MSM (44%). The main reasons given for not using it were "didn't think of it" (70%) and "trusting the partner" (15%). (Cf. graph 10)

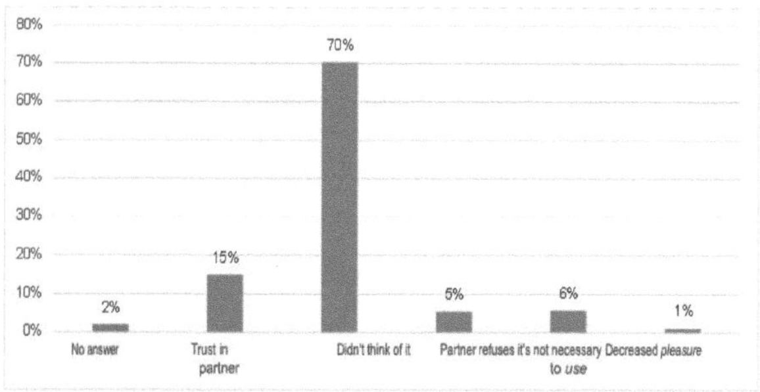

Graph 10: Breakdown of reasons for not using a condom at first sexual intercourse for all participants

Specifically, the rate of condom use at first sexual intercourse before the age of 15 (average age 13) was lower (21%), and even lower among boys (16%). The main reasons given for not using a condom at this age were that "I hadn't thought of it" (57%), "partner's refusal" (17%) and "I've never used a condom" (11%) (see graph 11).

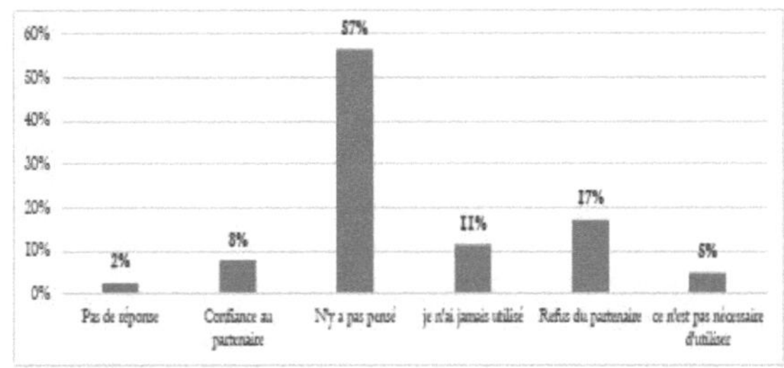

Figure 11: Breakdown of reasons for not using a condom a t first sexual intercourse before the age of 15

4.1.2. Frequency of intercourse

The frequency of sexual intercourse was assessed to better quantify the population's condom needs (see table 6).

Table 4: Average number of sexual encounters by sex and population type

Features	Average / days	Average/week	Interval/days
GENERAL POPULATION			
WOMAN			
15-24 years old	-	2	-
Aged 25-34	-	2	-
35-49 years old	-	2	-
50-64 years old	-	1	-
Total aged 15-64	-	2	-
MEN			
15-24 years old	-	3	-
Aged 25-34	-	3	-
35-49 years old	-	2	-
50-64 years old	-	2	-
Total aged 15-64	-	3	-
TOGETHER			
TOTAL aged 15-64	-	2	-
KEY POPULATION			
TS	6	42	3,3-8,7

MSM	2	14	1,6-3,2
UD	3	21	1,5-3,6
TG	3	21	1,2-4,3

In the general population, respondents reported having an average of two (02) sexual encounters per week. However, within the key populations, the average weekly number of sexual encounters was 42 for MSM, 14 for FSW and 21 for FSW and FSU.

4.1.3. Sexual relations at risk

When assessing sexual risk, the focus is on the last sexual encounter in the last 12 months (table 5).

Table 5: Condom use during last sexual intercourse in the general population

Features	Percentage reporting sexual intercourse in the last 12 months	Workforce	Percentage reporting sexual intercourse with a non-marital, non-cohabiting partner in the last 12 months last months	Workforce	Percentage reporting that a condom had been used during their last sexual intercourse with a non-marital, non-cohabiting partner	Workforce
WOMAN						
15-24 years old	90%	71	89%	63	41%	26
Aged 25-34	100%	83	57%	47	40%	19
35-49 years old	92%	23	30%	7	57%	4
Total women	95%	177	66%	117	42%	49
MEN						
15-24 years old	96%	120	89%	107	48%	51
Aged 25-34	97%	153	67%	103	53%	55
35-49 years old	100%	123	32%	39	64%	25
50-64 years old	80%	12	50%	6	50%	3
Total men	97%	408	63%	255	53%	134

TOGETHER 15-24 years old	94%	191	89%	170	45%	77
TOGETHER 25-64 years old	97%	394	51%	202	52%	106
TOGETHER 15-64 years	96%	585	64%	372	49%	183

Among the general population, 609 of the 615 participants declared their age. Of these 609 interviewees, 585 (96%) had had sexual intercourse during the last two years. 12 months, 372 (64%) of whom had had risky sex. Condom use during these risky sexual encounters was observed in 183 people (49%). Condom use during the last risky sexual encounter was even lower among female respondents aged 25-34 (40%) and 15-24 (41%).The reasons given for not using a condom during the last risky sexual encounter were dominated by "trusting your partner" (53%), "not having a partner" (12%) and "not using a condom" (12%). had not thought about it" (16%), "reduced pleasure" (10%) and "refusal of partner" (8%) (Cf. graph 12).

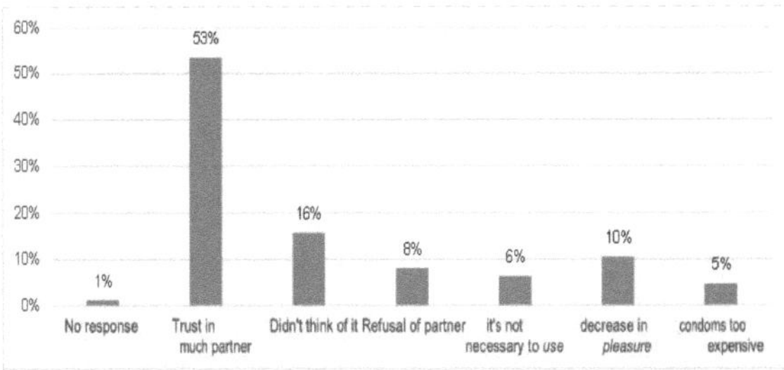

Figure 12: Comparison of orders and stock-outs between district pharmacies and wholesalers and semi-wholesalers

Among the key populations, condom use was found to be 92% among MSM, 75% among DU and 83% among MSM and TG (see graph 13).

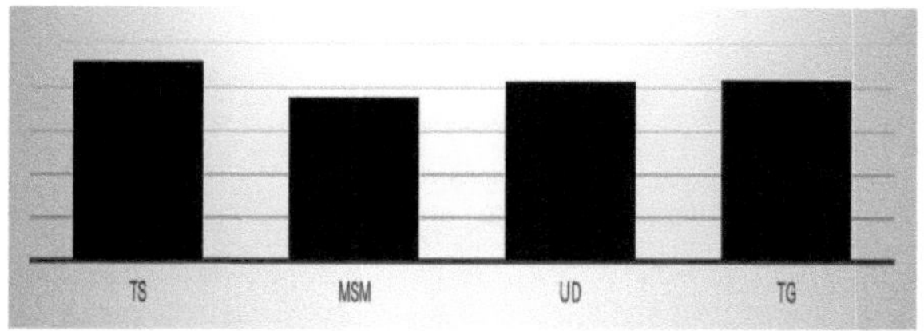

Graph 13: Rate of condom use during last high-risk sexual intercourse among key populations

4.1.4. Multi-partnership sexual

Multiple sexual partnerships were observed in 65% of men and 50% of women. Among female respondents, multiple sexual partnerships are high among 15-24 year olds (67%), with a declining trend with age until it disappears among those aged 50 and over. However, multi-partnering among male respondents remains consistently high (over 50%), higher than for women, with a slight drop in the 35-49 age group (49%).

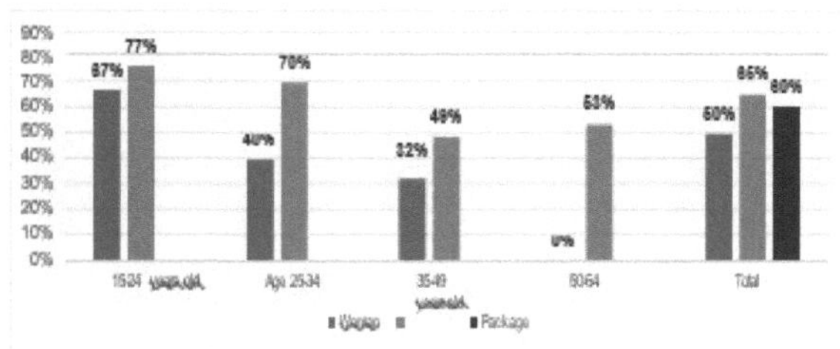

Figure 14: Percentage of respondents who have had more than one sexual partner in the last 12 months

4.2. Reasons for not using condoms

The reasons for not using condoms during risky sex are varied and the most recurrent were observed at two stages in the lives of the interviewees: at first sexual intercourse and at last sexual intercourse (Cf. graph15).

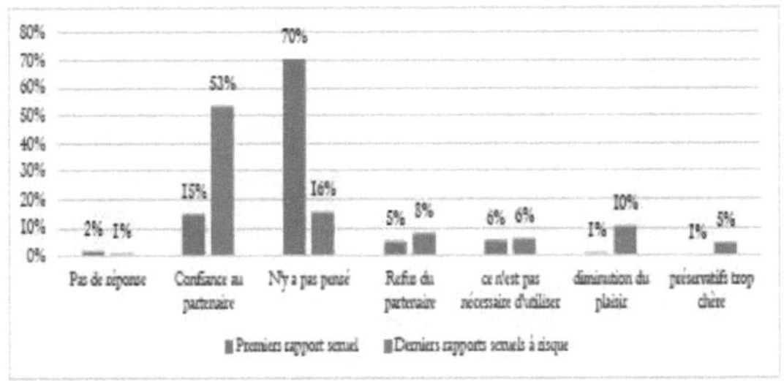

Figure 15: Change in reasons for not using a condom from first to last sexual intercourse

There has been an increase in reasons such as "trust in the partner", "less pleasure" and "condom too expensive", which rose from 15% to 53%, from 1% to 10% and from 1% to 5% respectively.However, the "didn't think of it" reason dropped from 70% to 16%.

4.3. Night-time supply of male condoms

Of the 1,707 people interviewed, 1,427 (84%) claimed to have access to condoms at night if they needed them. The highest rate was found among TS (91%) and the lowest among young teenagers aged 15-24 (67%) (see graph 14).

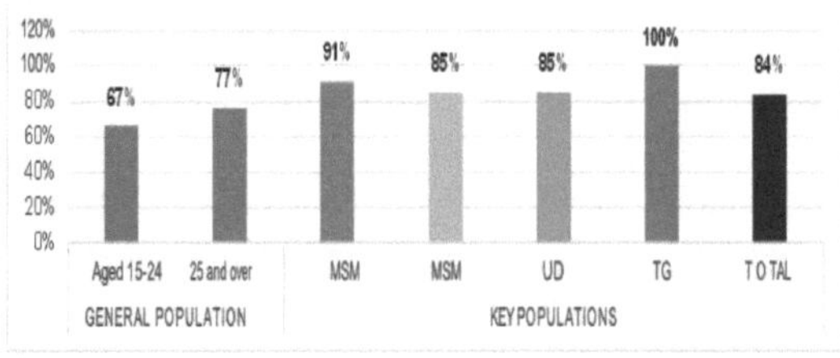

Graph 16: Percentage of participants with night-time access to condoms in case of need, by type of population

The points of sale to which the interviewees say they have access are shown in the graph below.

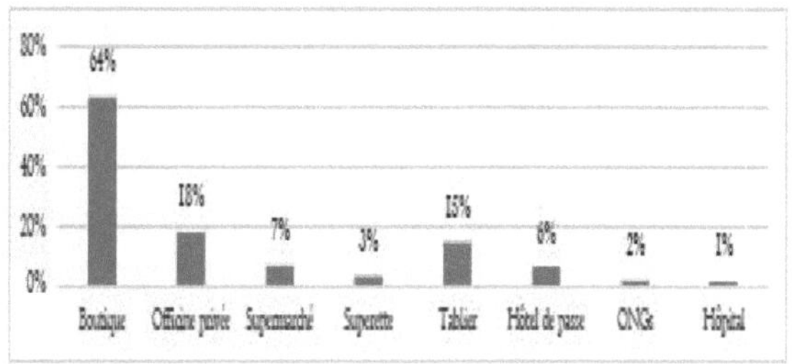

Graph 17: Percentage of participants with night-time access to condoms, by type of outlet

Respondents said they frequently had access to condoms at night if they needed them in shops (64%), private dispensaries (18%), aprons (15%) and brothels (6%).In addition, the male condom brands best known to participants are the most widely used. These are the PRUDENCE and COMPLICE brands from social marketing, the NO-LOGO free condoms and the KISS and DOMINO brands from the private sector (see chart 18).

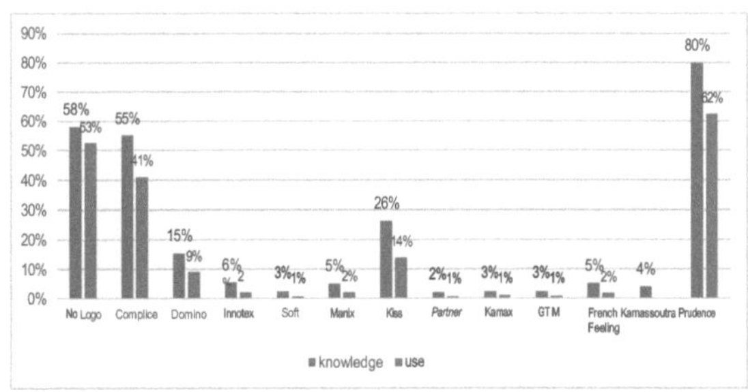

Graph 18: Percentage of participants aware of the condom brands offered and percentage using them

5. Knowledge of the female condom, lubricating gel and other types of condom

For the female condom and lubricating gel, three indicators were evaluated: "heard about", "knowledge" and "desire to use".

5.1. Female condom

A comparison of these indicators between the general population and key populations is shown in the graph below.

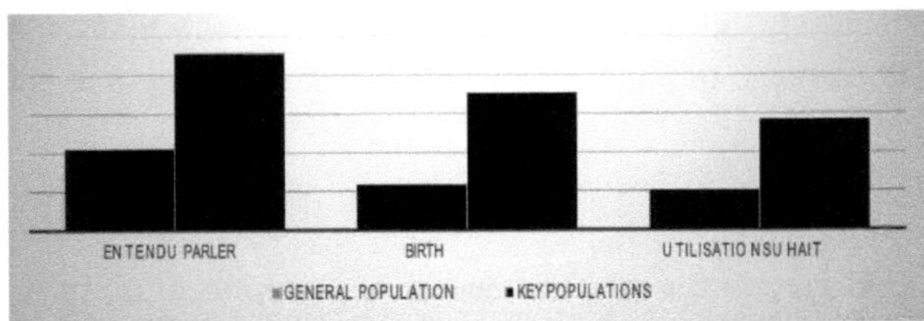

Graph 19: Comparison of female condom indicators between the general population and key populations

Of the 1,092 key populations interviewed, 915 (84%) had heard of the female condom, of whom 709 (77%) knew about it and 570 (62%) had not. would like to use it, compared with 422 (69%), 235 (56%) and 205 (49%) respectively in the general population.

5.2. Lubricating gel

For lubricant gels, of the 1,092 key populations interviewed, 977 (89%) have heard of them, including 938 (96%) who are aware of them and 905 (93%) who are not.would like to use it, compared with 338 (55%), 297 (88%) and 282 (83%) respectively for the general population (see chart 20).

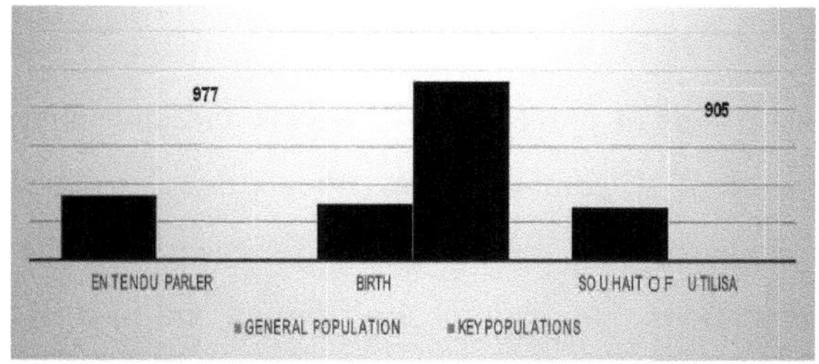

Graph 20: Comparison of indicators on lubricant gels between the general population and key populations

5.3. Other types of condom

In addition to male and female condoms, the evaluation covered other types of condom, such as the latex square and the finger pad, which very few participants had heard of (4% and 0.5% respectively).

V. DISCUSSIONS

Condom use as a means of preventing HIV, STIs and unwanted pregnancies is the main component of all combined prevention strategies aimed at controlling the HIV/AIDS epidemic. The main indicator for measuring the impact of our prevention interventions is condom use during the last high-risk sexual encounter (with a non-marital, non-cohabiting partner).In this study, there was a slight increase in this indicator in the general population, from 44.6% (Ciphia 2018) to 49.2% (ERUP 2021). In order to improve it, the fight must be directed at the obstacles to its use, which are of several kinds.

Reasons for non-use

At first intercourse, the rate of condom use is 30%, and the reasons for non-use are dominated by "didn't think of it" (70%) and "didn't know" (15%). "trust in the partner". Furthermore, when the first sexual intercourse took place before the age of 15, the rate of use was even lower (21%), with an average age of 13 and the same reasons for non-use ("hadn't thought of it" 57% and "didn't know" 57%)."17%). These reasons could be explained by ignorance of the risks and low exposure to awareness-raising messages, making it difficult to negotiate condom use. C. C. Y. Adohinzin, N. Meda, A. M. G. Belem, et al argue that this may be the consequence of social inequalities marked by the traditional and cultural preferences accorded to elders. Younger children, and especially girls, are generally deprived of information that is "considered sensitive" [4]. Similarly, communication strategies aimed at 10-14 year olds aim to equip them to know their bodies better, pay more attention to them and turn to sources of information on sexuality, but do not emphasise condom promotion. [18] Also, according to MacPhail [5], dominant social norms construct masculinity and profoundly affect the heterosexual experience of men. women. According to

Mazou [7], the difficulties young people have in accepting and using condoms are linked to the social environment in which they live and to the sudden nature of sexual intercourse in most cases. According to Gueilla [8], young people do not protect themselves because they often do not have a condom in their possession at the time of intercourse. The author explains this by the shame and disapproval adults feel towards adolescents when it comes to providing them with condoms.At the time of the last high-risk sexual encounter, the reasons given for not using a condom could be explained by an inadequate perception of the risk involved, or even a mistaken perception of the infected person, which is also seen as an obstacle to condom use by other authors [6;9]. For Ngamini [9], potential condom users must perceive HIV/AIDS as a real danger to their health, and also perceive the ravages of this disease in their immediate environment. Sarah's [6] study of HIV/AIDS prevention strategies in low- and middle-income countries seems to support this suggestion. For the author, campaigns focusing on sexual risk prevention have led to an increase in condom use over the last few decades. This is despite the fact that widespread condom use meets with cultural and religious resistance in some countries. Memmi S. and Orne-Gliemann J. point out that improving condom use by the general public could be achieved by focusing on interventions aimed at changing people's perceptions of social norms, knowledge about HIV/AIDS, self-efficacy and the effectiveness of condoms in protecting against HIV/AIDS [6].

Availability

In the public sector (free of charge), 16% (5) of district pharmacies did not place orders and 44% (12) of those who did place orders did not receive them. This led to stock-outs that lasted in average of 135 days. This shortfall in supply in the public sector can be explained by :

- Lack of ownership by stakeholders of the new measures for supplying condoms free of charge (district approach);

- Unfulfilled orders due to the relocation of condom stocks to the new Bouaké branch pending their redeployment to the districts covered by the branch;

- The shortages observed at wholesalers and semi-wholesalers are essentially due to the closure of international borders, which caused a delay in the supply of AIMAS products.

If people are to use condoms, the product must be readily available. This is confirmed by Memmi S. and Orne-Gliemann J., who state that condom use could be improved by focusing on availability [6].

Accessibility

The shops visited had a better permanent availability of condoms but were rarely open after midnight (56% of cases). On the other hand, the brothels had lower permanent availability than the shops, were all open after midnight (100% of cases, i.e. 24 hours a day) and were involved in the sale of no-logo condoms in 79% of cases. This finding highlights a market share that needs to be increased and reflects the inadequacy of the marketing plans of the various condom brands in the hotel sector.Hence the need to define standards for setting up condom sales outlets in the marketing-social and private sectors to ensure optimum accessibility.

Multi-partnership

According to the results, the younger the population, the more likely they are to have more than one sexual partner, reflecting their sexual vulnerability. This could be explained by :

- The fact that this young population is sexually active, has a desire for discovery, takes risks and is exposed to intergenerational sex in general;

- And more specifically by the fact that they have no source of income (girls aged 15-24), the desire to procreate and form a couple (women aged 25-49), and the affirmation of their masculinity (boys aged 15-24).

According to K Wood and R Jewkes, when negotiating their sexuality and the use of contraceptives, young girls said that they had been subjected to pressure and constraints from several sources to the point of not being able to make decisions as autonomous individuals [11]. According to Ngamini Ngui A, in Africa, in the social representation of contraception and HIV-AIDS prevention, girls are generally associated with the pill and boys with condoms. What's more, it's the boys who are more likely to take part in prevention campaigns and attend condom-use demonstrations. These observations are the result of gender inequalities and stereotypes [9].

For François Deniaud, this raises a symbolic dilemma. Condoms rationalise one of the most spontaneous acts of sex and love. Problematic elements come into play, such as the frustration of sexual pleasure, a feeling of self-deprecation, loss of identity and "waste" for the man when the condom containing his sperm is disposed of. There is also a feeling of guilt towards one's partner, who may be offended by the unilateral decision to use a condom, and a feeling of guilt towards one's elders, who may feel that they are flouting traditions, particularly the values of procreation and filiation, if they use a condom.

These feelings of guilt illustrate the symbolic threat of the condom to the individual and to society. Young people try to resolve their dilemmas in two ways: by trusting their partner, by refusing to use a condom or, at the extreme, by deliberately removing a condom during sexual intercourse before ejaculation; in the latter case, for example, the infectious risk of being contaminated by HIV (if consciously perceived) is taken in preference to the symbolic risk. not being able to enjoy and procreate, in other words, not being able to affirm one's gender and assume a social or sentimental role in the given context [11;12;13].

The limits of the study

A number of limitations need to be taken into account w h e n assessing the results. These include

• A number of biases may have influenced certain responses, including
Questions about sexual activity;
Difficulty remembering previous sexual activity;

• The methodological note was not submitted to the Ethics Committee for approval;

• As the survey was carried out in 30 towns and cities, the data cannot be extrapolated to the national level;

• Difficulty in mobilising financial resources to cover all the sentinel towns.

VI. RECOMMENDATIONS

CATEGORIES	FINDINGS	RECOMMENDATIONS	RESPONSIBLE ES
AVAILABIL ITE	Insufficient ownership of the new measures for supplying condoms free of charge (district approach)	Circulate the circular on the new arrangements for distributing free condoms Guiding players Supervise the trained players	PNLS
	Unfulfilled or partially fulfilled customer orders direct	Follow up orders	PNLS
	Stock-outs of condoms observed among wholesalers and semi-wholesalers	Organise quarterly supply and distribution monitoring meetings	GTT-CPP
	Absence of private sector distribution in 5 out of 18 towns and social marketing in 2. cities out of 18		
ACCESSIBIL ITE	No-logo condoms (free) available at points of sale	- Branding free condoms	PNLS
	Presence of smuggled condom brands on the market	Implementation of activities relating to the regulation and control of condoms and lubricant gels	DR/DD
teenager under 15	first sexual intercourse before the age of 15 occurred on average at the age of 13, with 21% condom use rate	develop awareness-raising messages tailored to the 10-14 age group readapting awareness-raising messages for the target audience to the realities of the moment	PNLS
	Inadequate perception of the risks involved Low exposure to awareness messages Difficulties in negotiating condom use		
Frequency of sexual intercourse	key populations have an average of : FS: 42 sexual encounters MSM: 14 sexual encounters FSU: 21 sexual encounters TG: 21 sexual encounters	review condom supplies incorporate the new staffing standards into the document setting out standards and procedures for the distribution of condoms and lubricant gels	PNLS
Last sexual intercourse (general population)	49% condom use rate a lack of risk perception ; the existence of prejudices about condoms;	step up condom promotion to deconstruct prejudices about condoms	PNLS

CATEGORIES	FINDINGS	RECOMMENDATIONS	RESPONSIBLE
	the desire to form a couple and the desire to have children		
multi-sex partnership	women's multiple sexual partnerships are high (67%) in the 15-24 age group, declining with age to reach zero in the 50+ age group and over	Intensify awareness-raising campaigns on the risks of multi-partnership and on the promotion of the correct wearing and use of protective clothing. systematic use of condoms	PNLS
	the number of sexual partners is consistently high (over 80%) in men of all ages		
Reasons for not using condoms	A lack of awareness of the risks involved	revise awareness-raising messages with an emphasis on the pauci-symptomatic or asymptomatic STIs and HIV	PNLS
	Condom costs out of control	include condoms in the room kits of the hotels where you stay	PNLS
		install automatic condom dispensers in hot spots	GTT-CCP AIMAS
Female condom	low awareness among the general population insufficient availability insufficient promotion	promote the female condom encourage social marketing of female condoms	GTT-CPP
Lubricating gels	People's need for lubricating gels	social marketing of lubricant gels	GTT-CPP

CONCLUSION

This study shows that the rate of condom use during risky sex in the general population remains low (less than 50%). Obstacles to use include the reasons for non-use, inadequate risk perception, intergenerational sex and inadequate availability of condoms. There is therefore an urgent need to step up awareness and information campaigns, while adapting their content to the real needs of the target populations, so as to pass on to them the skills required for effective prevention, particularly as regards condom use.However, the issue of correct and systematic condom use should not be overlooked. Adolescent sexuality is often spontaneous, new and highly emotional, and may also be tinged with a degree of shame and secrecy. In this social and behavioural context, condoms may not be used correctly or may even be ignored by both partners [17].This concern is reflected in the results of the PSI survey [15], which showed that of the 74.0% of young people who thought they were capable of using condoms correctly, only 21.7% had successfully gone through the five stages of condom use. This is an important factor that can positively influence young people's personal decision to use condoms systematically during sex. So it is not enough to make condoms available; it is essential to make their use efficient, by training potential users in how to use them [4].Although there is a problem of availability, it would be preferable, in the interests of offering a differentiated service tailored to the needs of the target populations, to conduct a CAP (knowledge, practical skills) study on correct condom use.

BIBLIOGRAPHY

1. Plan Stratégique National de lutte contre le VIH, le sida et les infections sexuellement transmissibles 2021-2025; 2021; PNLS; p41.

2. Background note on the position statement on condoms and the prevention of HIV, other sexually transmitted infections and unintended pregnancies; July 2015; UNAIDS.

3. Rapport de l'analyse situationnelle des préservatifs et gels lubrifiants dans le cadre de l'approche du marché total; 2021; PNLS. P10.

4. C. C. Y. Adohinzin, N. Meda, A. M. G. Belem, et al. Male condom use: knowledge, attitudes and skills of young people in Burkina Faso. S.F.S.P. | "Santé Publique". 2017/1 Vol. 29 | pages 95 to 103.

5. MacPhail C and Campbell C. I think condoms are good but, aai, I hate those things': condom use among adolescents and young people in a Southern African township. Social Science & Medicine. 2001; 52(11):1613-1627. Doi: 10.1016/S0277-9536(00)00272-0.

6. Desgrées du Loû A, Memmi S, Orne-Gliemann J. Strategies of HIV Prevention in Low and Middle-Income Countries. The Open Infectious Diseases Journal. 010;4:92-100. Electronic publication date 15/9/2010. Doi: 10.2174/1874279301004010092.

7. Mazou G. Sexual risk behaviour of schoolchildren: an analysis of the social determinants of condom 27 non-use among students at the Lycée moderne II in Bouaké. European Scientific Journal. 2014;10(2):128 p.

8. Gueilla G. Santé Sexuelle et de la Reproduction des Jeunes au Burkina Faso: Un état des lieux. New York: Alan Guttmacher Institute; 2004. 37 p.

9. Ngamini Ngui A, Determinants of condom use among young people in Côte d'Ivoire. Médecine d'Afrique Noire. 2010;57(4): S41-S135.

10. Lacombe E. The condom: questions and answers. Le Médecin du Québec. 2006;41(2):37-69.

11. K Wood, R Jewkes. Issues in Reproductive Health. 2012;(3):80-91

12. DENIAUD F. (991) "Sida, préservatifs et jeunesse urbaine en Côte-d'Ivoire: un essai d'ethnoprévention", Bulletin de liaison du CNDT, special issue, pp.46-69.

13. GINOUX-POUYAUD C. (1992) "Etude sociologique sur le choix du partenaire sexuel chez les femmes en âge de procréer à Koumassi et Marcory", Bulletin du GIDIS-CI, 2, p.42

14. DEDY S. et TAPE G. (1991) Comportements sexuels et sida en Côte-d'Ivoire (Rapport préliminaire), PNLS, Abidjan. (1992) "Les comportements sexuels à risque en Côte-d'Ivoire", Bulletin du OlDIS-CI, 2, pp.63- 72.

15. Population service international (PSI). Enquête de base pour suivre et analyser les déterminants de l'utilisation consistente du condom en vue de prévenir le VIH/Sida au sein de la population générale. Burkina Faso: PSI; 2009. p20.

16. Audrey P, Katie O, MacPhail C, William C. Earliness of sexual debut and associated HIV risk factors in young people. women and men in South Africa. International Perspectives on Sexual and Reproductive Health. 2010;Special Issue:29-37.

17. Johannes B, Sybille T, Brigitte F. Contraception among adolescents. Forum Med Suisse. 2006;6:1004-10.

18. Behaviour change communication strategy for HIV and AIDS in côte d'ivoire 2016 - 2020. Version 2018.PNLS; p42.

A. Need for male condoms and quantities distributed by sentinel city by total market segment (distribution 2021)

sentinel cities	NEEDS	Districts	referral hospitals e	TOTAL FREE E	AIMAS	PRIVATE	TOTAL X
BONDOUKOU	1 033 253	2 575 800	6 600	2 582 400	196 740	0	2 779 140
BOUAKE	2 268 387	492 200	2 900	495 100	1 334 790	157 012	1 986 902
SOUBRE	1 504 861	199 100	10 200	209 300	1 696 740	0	1 906 040
DALOA	1 865 328	160 200	173 700	333 900	1 305 720	236 769	1 876 389
ABENGOUROU	1 155 883	173 600	155 600	329 200	1 344 540	0	1 673 740
GAGNOA	1 958 106	48 000	12 000	60 000	1 171 590	172 800	1 404 390
SAN-PEDRO	1 889 647	43 900	8 000	51 900	1 238 220	15 234	1 305 354
ADZOPE	664 808	51 000	15 000	66 000	1 006 500	0	1 072 500
DUEKOUE	1 316 622	64 600	12 000	76 600	799 140	0	875 740
AGBOVILLE	977 247	12 000	0	12 000	815 610	0	827 610
BOUAFLE	1 335 682	2 900	9 600	12 500	711 330	0	723 830
GUIGLO	546 815	78 200	0	78 200	602 250	0	680 450
SEGUELA	610 357	121 200	15 200	136 400	475 530	0	611 930
DIVO	1 220 233	65 200	144 900	210 100	397 770	0	607 870
DAOUKRO	573 526	29 600	10 000	39 600	400 620	0	440 220
ISSIA	948 970	18 600	136 900	155 500	178 350	0	333 850
YAMOUSSOUKR O	1 301 671	28 000	32 400	60 400	259 380	0	319 780
TABOU	594 207	59 000	8 000	67 000	232 650	0	299 650
MANKONO	692 779	7 200	13 400	20 600	98 370	0	118 970
AGNIBILEKR	553 563	38 000	19 400	57 400	28 500	0	85 900

OU							
KANI	216 626	33 700	8 500	42 200	19 200	0	61 400
KATIOLA	362 479	31 200	500	31 700	20 730	0	52 430
BEOUMI	462 421	41 600	400	42 000	5 850	0	47 850
SAKASSOU	287 699	38 300	3 500	41 800	1 350	0	43 150
TOUBA	269 712	11 400	8 800	20 200	0	0	20 200
BUYO	507 239	15 400	1 600	17 000	0	0	17 000
OUME	926 940	15 600	0	15 600	0	0	15 600
KOUNAHIRI	229 414	13 500	0	13 500	0	0	13 500
OUANINOU	165 993	5 000	3 600	8 600	0	0	8 600
KORO	197 034	7 500	0	7 500	0	0	7 500

B. QUESTIONNAIRES

AVAILABILITY GRID

Health region:

Health district:

Location:

Company name:

Type of business :wholesaler semi-wholesaler

PRODUCT SUPPLY	O UI	NO N	OBSERVA TI ON
1. Have you placed any orders in the last 06 months?			
2. If not, why not			
3. if yes, specify the structure or other sources of supply			
4. Were these orders filled? If not, why not?			
STORAGE MANAGEMENT			
5. Have you experienced any break-ups in the last six months?			
6. If yes, why?			
7. Duration of the break	...	days	
8. What steps have you taken?			
STORAGE CONDITIONS	O UI	NO N	OBSERVA TI ON
9. the shop is cleaned periodically (see cleaning schedule)			
10. the condoms are stored in a humidity-free, well-lit room, and well ventilated			
11. condoms are protected from direct sunlight			
12. the depot is protected from water leaks			
13. The depot has fire-fighting equipment			
14. Depot staff know how to use fire-fighting equipment			
15. Has and knows how to use fire-fighting equipment			
16. condoms areDisposed away from electric motors and lights fluorescent			
17. Restricts access to the shop to authorised personnel (make sure condoms are kept in a locked place)			
18. boxes of condoms and lubricant gels are stacked at least 10 centimetres from the floor, 30 centimetres from walls and other stacks, and 2.5 metres high maximum			For district
19. boxes of condoms and lubricant gels are storedon suitable storage equipment			For wholesalers/ emi-wholesalers

	AVAILABILITY Y/N	REMPLISSAGE (Updated) Y/N	comments
20. Condoms and lubricating gels are stored in a place protected from insecticides, pesticides and other contaminants. chemicals, flammables, hazardous materials, old files, office supplies and other equipment			
21. Condoms and lubricating gels are stored in such a way as to make them easy to remove. First Out of Date - First Out" (FOPOF) principle and stock management			
22. The boxes of condoms and gel lubricants are arranged so that the arrows point upwards, and that the identification labels, expiry dates and production dates are clearly visible			
23. damaged or out-of-date condoms and lubricant gels are separated from stocks currents			
24. Respect the procedures in force concerning their destruction (existence of the PPI destruction procedures manual/integrated SIGL manual)			

TOOLS	AVAILABILITY Y/N	REMPLISSA GE (Updated) Y/N	comments
DISTRICT PHARMACY			
25. Stock sheet			
26. Delivery and transfer note			
27. ARV, IO* dispensing register			
28. Monthly ARV dispensing report, IO*.			
29. Monthly Order Report - ARV, IO			
30. Complaints booklet			
31. Expiry date tracking table			
32. Inventory sheet of unusable condoms			
WHOLESALER AND ½ WHOLESALER			
33. Order forms			
34. Delivery notes			
35. Stock management software			

ACCESSIBILITY EVALUATION GRID

Health region:.

Health district:

Location:

Type of outlet

<table>
<tr><td>

Is it a hot spot

Yes | No   No | __|

</td></tr>
</table>

Shop : | |

Private practice: | |

Supermarket: | |

Superette : | |

Apron : | |

Hotel : | |

Vending machines : | |

Other | specify:

Working days/days/week

Opening hours : | || Hours | Minutes | Minutes

Closing time : | || Time| Minutes

CONDOMS AVAILABLE

MODE OF SUPPLY		Sales depot	
		Pay Cash	
		On credit	
DO YOU ALWAYS HAVE CONDOMS AVAILABLE DURING BUSINESS HOURS?		YES	
		NO	
IF NOT, WHO DO YOU BUY FROM?		stock at home	
		use of a colleague	
		recourse to distribution	
TOTAL MARKET SEGMENT	BRANDS	PRESENCE	
		YES	NO
PUBLIC SECTOR	No logo		
SOCIAL MARKETING SECTOR	Partner		
	Caution		
PRIVATE SECTOR	Domino		
	Innotex		
	Soft		
	Manix		
	Kiss		
	Partner		
	Kamax		
	GTM		
	French Feelings		
	Kamassutra		
	Other (please specify)		
	Other (please specify)		
	Other (please specify)		

EVALUATION GRID FOR USE

Health region:

Health district:

Location:

Date of interview: | || | || | |||

SOCIO-DEMOGRAPHIC SITUATION

1. TYPE OF POPULATION

TS: | | MSM: | | DU: | | TG: | | General population: ||

2. Age : ||Years

3. Sex : ||

4. WHAT IS THE HIGHEST LEVEL OF EDUCATION YOU HAVE ACHIEVED:

Preschool: | |

Primary: | |

Secondary: | |

Superior | |

Don't know : | |

Refusal: | |

SEXUAL BEHAVIOUR

I would now like to ask you a few questions about your sexual activity in order to gain a better understanding of some of life's problems. The information you provide will remain strictly confidential and will not be divulged to anyone. If I ask a question that you don't want to answer, just let me know and I'll move on to the next question. If you need to clarify any questions, please let me know. (Check the presence of other people. Before continuing, make sure you are in private with the person being interviewed) vaginal intercourse, anal intercourse; oral intercourse

1. AT WHAT AGE DID YOU HAVE SEXUAL INTERCOURSE FOR THE VERY FIRST TIME? If answer 00 ð stop questionnaire	Never had sex ... 00 in years years...1 don't know8
2. THE FIRST TIME YOU HAD SEXUAL INTERCOURSE, WAS A CONDOM USED?	Yes1 No2 Can't remember 8
3. IN THE LAST 12 MONTHS, HAVE YOU HAD SEXUAL INTERCOURSE? If answer 2 ð Q17	Yes 1 No 2
4. WHEN DID YOU LAST HAVE SEXUAL INTERCOURSE?	.... days ago 1 .... weeks ago2 .... months ago.3
5. WHAT WAS YOUR RELATIONSHIP WITH THE PERSON WITH WHOM YOU LAST HAD SEXUAL INTERCOURSE? Insist that the answer refers to the type of relationship at the time of intercourse If 'boyfriend', ask: LIVETOGETHER AS IF YOUWERE MARRIED? If 'yes', circle '2'. If 'no', circle '3'.	Spouse 1 Partner cohabiting 2 Boyfriend3 partner occasional 4 client.. 5 Other(please specify)6
6. THE LAST TIME THAT YOU WERE HAVE SEXUAL RELATIONS, HAS A CONDOM BEEN USED?	Yes1
HAS IT BEEN USED?	No 2
7. IF NO, WHY NOT	Trusting your partner
	It is not necessary to use
	I've never used
	Religious beliefs
	Does not like condoms
	Reduced pleasure
	Didn't have a condom in the room
	Partner refusal
	Condoms not available in the shop
	Condoms too expensive
	We used a other contraceptive
	Didn't think of it
	To get pregnant

	No answer
8. HOW OLD IS THIS PERSON? If DK, insist : HOW OLD IS THIS PERSON?	Age of sexual partner DK 98
9. IN THE LAST 12 MONTHS, HAVE YOU HAD SEXUAL INTERCOURSE WITH ANOTHER PERSON?If answer 2 ð Q 14	Yes 1 No 2
10. DURING SEX WITH THIS OTHER PERSON WAS A CONDOM BEEN USED?	Yes 1 No 2
11. WHICH IS YOUR RELATIONSHIP WITH THIS PERSON? Insist that the answer refers to the type of relationship at the time of intercourse If 'boyfriend', ask: LIVE TOGETHER AS IF YOU MARRIED? If 'yes', circle '2'. If 'no', circle '3'.	Spouse 1 Partner cohabiting2 Boyfriend3 partner occasional4 client.........5 Other(please specify) 6
12. HOW OLD IS THIS PERSON?	Age of sexual partner
If don't know, insist : APPROXIMATELY HOW OLD IS THIS PERSON?	DK 98
13. APART FROM THESE TWO PEOPLE, HAVE YOU HAD	Yes 1
FROM REPORTS SEXWITH A OTHER	No 2
ANYONE IN THE LAST 12 MONTHS?	
If answer 2 => Q15	
14. WAS A CONDOM USED?	Yes 1 No 2
15. NUMBER OF SEXUAL ENCOUNTERS (General population)	/WEEK/ MONTH
16.HOW MANY SEXUAL PARTNERS COULD YOU HAVE PER DAY? (Reserved for key populations)	Number of partners MAXIMUM : MINIMUM :
17. NAME FIVE (05) BRANDS OF CONDOMS THAT YOU	1 :
DO YOU KNOW IT?	2 :
	3 :
	4 :
	5 :
18. NAME THREE (03) BRANDS OF CONDOMS THAT	1 :
DO YOU USE REGULARLY?	2 :
	3 :
19. IN CASE OF NEED, DO YOU MANAGE TO OBTAIN CONDOMS DURING THE NIGHT?	YES NO
20. IF YES, WHERE YOU GET THESE	Shop

CONDOMS?			Private practice
			Supermarket
			Supermarket
			Apron
			Hotel
			Vending machines
			Other specify
21. HOW EVALUATE-YOU PRESERVATIVE ? (during the day)	ACCESS	AUX	Very easy
			Fairly easy
			Neutral
			Not very difficult
			Very difficult
22. HOW EVALUATE YOU PRESERVATIVE ? (during the night)	ACCESS	AUX	Very easy
			Fairly easy
			Neutral
			Not very difficult
			Very difficult
23. HAVE YOU HEARD OF THE FEMALE CONDOM? IF 2=> Q 21			Yes1 No2
24. ARE YOU FAMILIAR WITH THE FEMALE CONDOM?the participant must be able to describe the female condom			Yes1 No2
25. WOULD YOU LIKE TO USE A A FEMALE CONDOM?			Yes1 No 2
26. WHAT OTHER TYPES OF CONDOM HAVE YOU HEARD OF?			SQUAREFROM LATEX...1 DOIGTIER....2 OTHER (please specify) 3
27. HAVE YOU HEAR SPEAK ABOUT WATER-BASED LUBRICATING GELS? IF 2=> end of questionnaire			Yes 1 No2
28. ARE YOU FAMILIAR WITH WATER-BASED LUBRICATING GELS? the participant must be able to describe the presentation (sachet or dosette / tube)			Yes1 No2
29. WOULD YOU LIKE TO USE WATER-BASED LUBRICATING GELS?			Yes1 No2
30. DO YOU KNOW A PLACE WHERE PEOPLE CAN BUY LUBRICATING GELS?			Yes1 No2
31. HOW DO YOU RATE ACCESS TO GELS? LUBRICANTS (during the day) ?			Very easy
			Fairly easy
			Neutral
			Not very difficult
			Very difficult

32. HOW DO YOU RATE ACCESS TO GELS? LUBRICANTS (overnight)	Very easy
	Fairly easy
	Neutral
	Not very difficult
	Very difficult

C. BREAKDOWN OF CONDOM BRANDS BY SALES OUTLET

	no logo	accomplice	domino	innotex	caution	manix	kiss	partner	kamax	gtm	french feeling	kamasoutra	soft	protector	condoms	herosound	livex	today
Shops	15	36			49		11			2			1	4	5	1	2	
Aprons	7	10			6		6							1	1	1		
Pass hotels	10	2			6			1	1	1								
Coffee kiosks		1																
tobacco shop		1		1														
Distributors automatic		1		1														
Private practices		3	6	2	4	4	6		2	2		3	3					
Supermarket	1			1			1									1		1
Maquis		1		1			1											
Bistro	1			1														

A. DATA COLLECTION SHEET

		QUANTITY	January	February	March	April	May	June	S1 total	rate of satisfaction	rate of distribution
		DATA COLLECTION GRID FOR CONDOMS 2021									
		LOCALITY:									
Health District	Condoms	Ordered	0	0	0	0	0	0	0	#DIV/0!	
		Received	0	0	0	0	0	0	0		
		Distributed	0	0	0	0	0	0	0		#DIV/0!
		SDU	0	0	0	0	0	0	0		
	Lubricating gels	Ordered	0	0	0	0	0	0	0	#DIV/0!	
		Received	0	0	0	0	0	0	0		
		Distributed	0	0	0	0	0	0	0		#DIV/0!
		SDU	0	0	0	0	0	0	0		
NAME of wholesaler or 1/2 wholesaler:	Condoms	Ordered							0	#DIV/0!	
		Received							0		
		Distributed							0		#DIV/0!
		SDU							0		
	Lubricating gels	Ordered							0	#DIV/0!	
		Received							0		
		Distributed							0		#DIV/0!
		SDU							0		
	Condoms	Ordered							0	#DIV/0!	
		Received							0		
		Distributed							0		#DIV/0!
		SDU							0		
	Condoms	Ordered							0	#DIV/0!	
		Received							0		
		Distributed							0		#DIV/0!
		SDU							0		

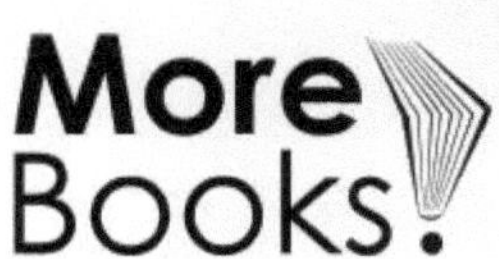

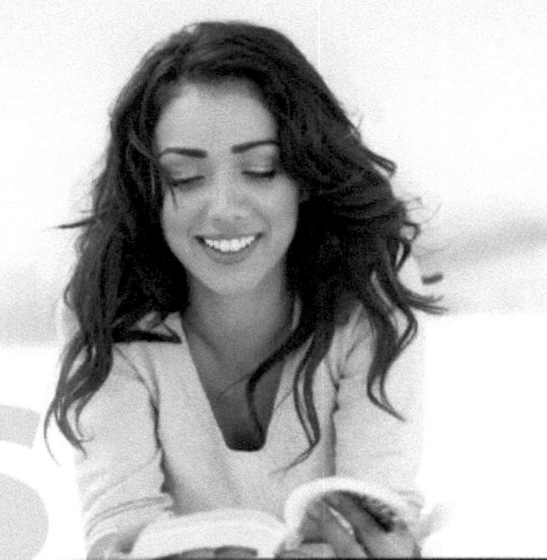

Buy your books fast and straightforward online - at one of world's fastest growing online book stores! Environmentally sound due to Print-on-Demand technologies.

Buy your books online at
www.morebooks.shop

Kaufen Sie Ihre Bücher schnell und unkompliziert online – auf einer der am schnellsten wachsenden Buchhandelsplattformen weltweit! Dank Print-On-Demand umwelt- und ressourcenschonend produziert.

Bücher schneller online kaufen
www.morebooks.shop

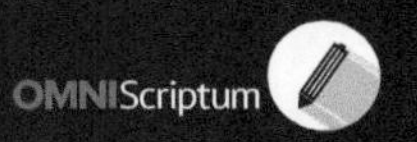

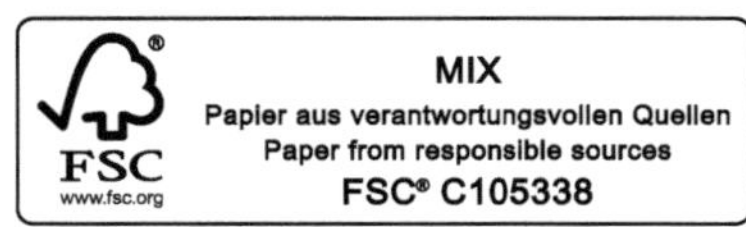

Printed by Books on Demand GmbH, Norderstedt / Germany